Comprehensive
Diabetes Guide

Comprehensive Diabetes Guide

An Informative Book.

Grace Ampofoh

To order additional copies of this book, contact:
Xlibris
844-714-8691
www.Xlibris.com
Orders@Xlibris.com
842185

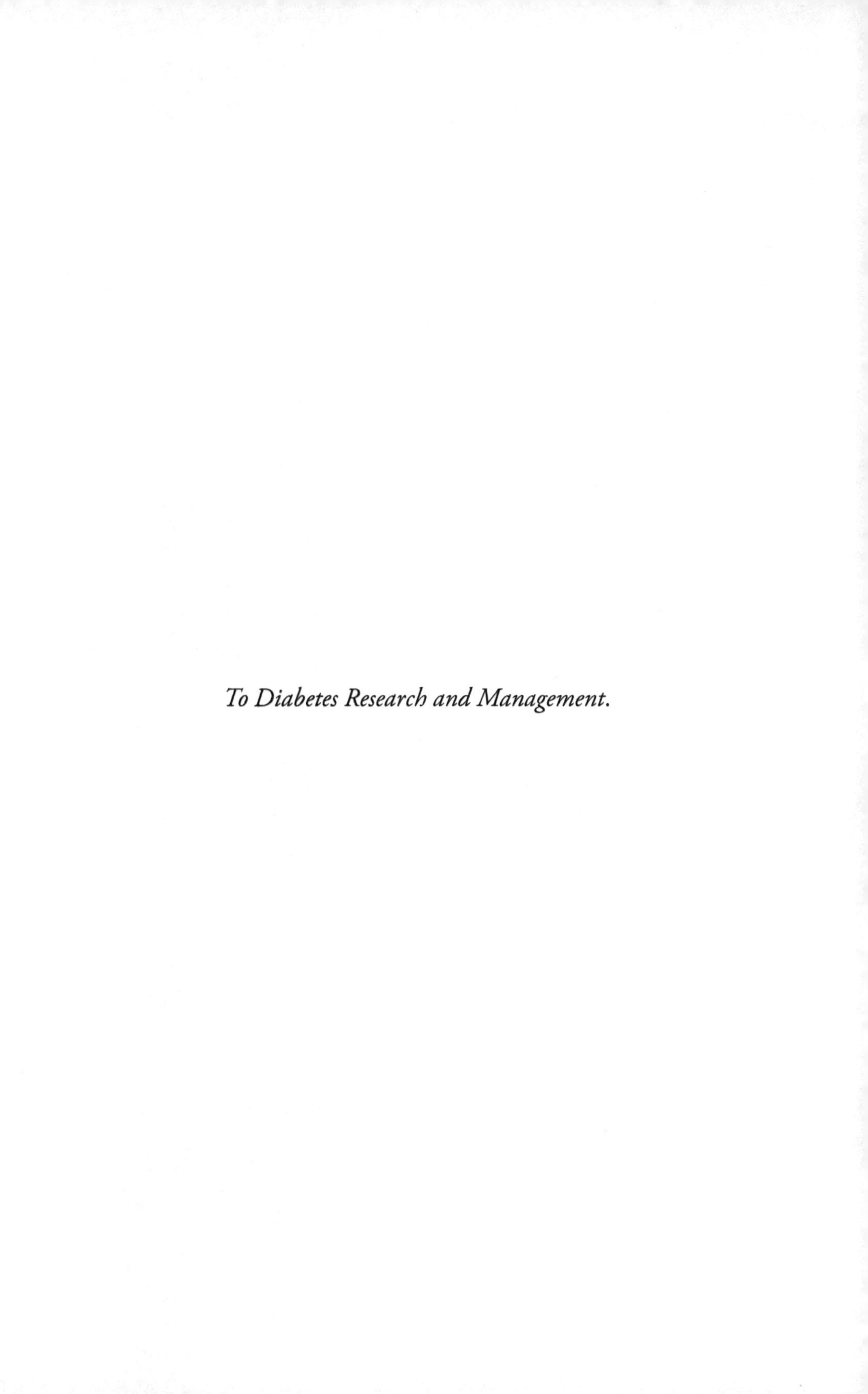

To Diabetes Research and Management.

Acknowledgements

My sincere thanks goes to the Publishers for their assistance.

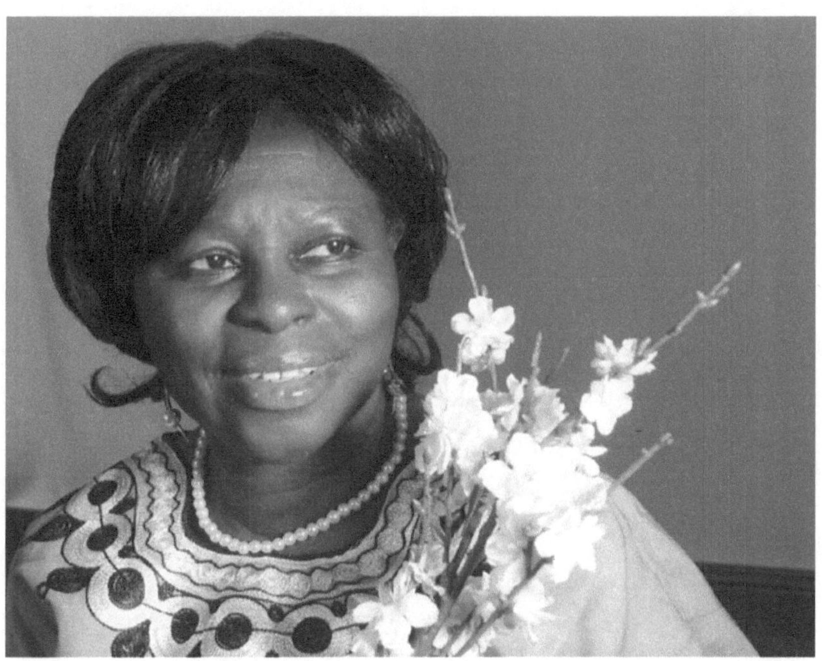

I also thank my family and friends for their
support. I owe a debt of gratitude to
the experts in the globe who continue to research hard to
promote awareness of diabetes, treatment modality, and self-care
management of diabetes. Lastly, I thank God for his grace.

TABLE OF CONTENTS

CHAPTER 1

INTRODUCTION

During her long period of nursing career, Author Grace Atea Ampofoh took care of many elderly diabetic patients, including family members. "Comprehensive Diabetes Guide" is a book written not only for her legacy, but also for her contribution to worldwide campaigns for diabetes research and awareness of the disease, as well as diabetes self-care management. Updates of current reports and information as related to diabetes have been highlighted in this health resource guide. To achieve and maintain a healthy lifestyle as a diabetic, Atea Ampofoh added that self- management of diabetes is imperative. She said, "Just because you've been diagnosed with diabetes does not mean your life cannot be a wonderful and exciting journey." The author had long experience in Gerontology, and she worked hard daily as a Registered Nurse, and as a diabetic patient herself. So, she understood and learned to be an advocate, a champion, who has been working wholeheartedly to raise awareness of diabetes. **The author** challenges her audience, diabetics and health-care providers to work closely with **each other for successful outcome. Regarding management of all types of diabetes, medical supervision by routine doctors' visits is necessary. Based on the laboratory tests' results, the doctor can evaluate how the patient is handling the disease throughout the journey to recovery. The doctor can change medications or adjust medication**

doses, to control high blood glucose levels to normal range. A diabetic patient can be referred to diabetes management classes with various health-care personnel, including dietician for diet control, fitness center for exercise and weight control. Government programs such as Medicare and Medicaid are utilized for financial assistance. Everyone plays a role in the society to support diabetes management globally. Diabetes is a condition that you must just live with longer and take good care of managing your disease, and your health in general. Although this might be hard, time consuming, and requires the help of loved- ones, health- care team and the society in general. It is hard, but it is a choice you have to make for your survival. **Comparatively,** it is not easy either, for example, an epileptic individual to live with this illness in life, and that he or she has to suffer from the negative impact, emotionally and physically in some cultures. In fact, Diabetes must not slowly get worse or control your life, because if you have diabetes, you have to be in charge of living a healthy lifestyle. You can control prediabetes from slowly reaching Type-2 diabetes, and Type-2 from getting to complications of diabetes, including heart disease, stroke, nerve damage, eye disease, and kidney disease. **Today, there is hope and more opportunity for diabetics than a hundred years ago. More research workers have tried to develop new plans for diabetes management, such as home management education, diabetics with complication of kidney disease can receive kidney transplant treatment or dialysis, and even both. Wow! Same individuals living with diabetes can live longer because of these interventions.**

CHAPTER 2

WORLD HEALTH ORGANIZATION {WHO}- Report Update

WORLD HEALTH ORGANIZATION {WHO} –Updates of diabetes mellitus global awareness- {Bing.com}.

Aside from Coronavirus-19, experts from the World Health Organization {WHO} also warn that diabetes is an emerging pandemic. Diabetes is a chronic condition that requires medical attention. Some of the goals we need to focus on are:

1. Promoting healthy diets globally.
2. Preventing and controlling non-communicable diseases like diabetes.
3. Creating health promotion, fitness and workshop centers.
4. Encourage multimedia Education.
5. Access to diabetes treatment and management are encouraged with medical supervision.

Diabetes overview on 10/8/2021.- World Health Organization:

Diabetes is a chronic disease that occurs either when the pancreas does not produce enough insulin, or when the body cannot effectively use insulin it produces. Insulin is a hormone that regulates blood sugar or glucose. Hyperglycemia/ raised blood sugar is a common effect of uncontrolled diabetes and over time leads to serious damage to many of the body's systems, especially the nerves and blood vessels. In 2014, 85% of adults aged 18 years and older had diabetes.

Global report on diabetes- World Health Organization:

Diabetes is a serious chronic disease that occurs either when the pancreas does not produce enough insulin {a hormone that regulates blood sugar or glucose}, or when the body cannot effectively use the insulin it produces. Diabetes is an important public health problem.

World Health Organization report on Diabetes in Western Pacific.

On 5/5/2021 Report: Diabetes is a chronic disease that occurs either when the pancreas does not produce enough of the blood sugar – regulating hormone insulin or when the body cannot effectively use the insulin it produces. Hyperglycemia / elevated blood sugar is common effect of diabetes that eventually leads to serious damage to many of the body's system, especially, the nerves and blood vessels. Diabetes is one of the four major non communicable diseases. About 131 million / 8.4% people in the Western Pacific Region had diabetes in 2014. {https:// www.who.int/westernpacific/health-topics/diabetes}

CHAPTER 3

DIABETES RESEARCH REPORT

The author talks about her personal experiences and shares with her audience as a story teller. Ampofoh said, "Diabetic individuals have the opportunity to write their own story joyfully, with expected outcome for the future generation". The author continued by saying, "Not too long ago, in July 2019, I watched a C-SPAN program U.S.A. on the television. It was a forum of panel debate on DIABETES RESEARCH REPORT".

I want to share what I learned with the readers, because the program was educational. Kidney transplant research has successfully been done to improve kidney disease treatment. Advance in technology has increased, and complication of diabetes has declined. New treatment by using autoimmune factor and stem cell to initiate treatment seems to work faster. Children diagnosed with Type-1 diabetes were among the participants.

I want to share some of the information with my audience for encouragement. So, one participant who was diagnosed with Type-1 diabetes at the age eight, has improved due to advancement of treatment modalities. Now she is seventeen years old, and she is even an active musician. Another participant who was diagnosed with Type-1 diabetes was just three years old. He is now a successful student. He plays tennis, enjoys golf and water sports.

One speaker, a U.S. senator, and a member of Special Aging Committee, encouraged us to focus on the need to reduce the cause of INSULIN. He added that a new special diabetes program is signed into law in the U.S. senate.

Another member from the U.S. senate said, Artificial pancreas treatment is used in my state in Nevada, U.S.A. Don't ignore the economic burden on you and your family, if you are a diabetic and even the high demand on society as a whole. Why do I worry about this as a diabetic? It is overwhelming to imagine a diabetic patient and the family dealing about how to handle the disease. Not only that health- care systems suffer financially, considering insurers, and government programs like Medicare and Medicaid try to balance their budget to pay hospital bills, medication, doctors, and the need to pay for various outpatient therapies for even one individual.

My take is:

All the positive things I learned from the C-SPAN - Diabetes Research Report, as a Registered Nurse living with diabetes empowered me to prepare myself to join the "World Health Organization{WHO}" by writing books to raise awareness of diabetes and diabetes self- care management for today in the midst of COVID-19 PANDEMIC outbreak. What about future generation living with diabetes? A word to the wise is enough. What challenged me was the final report given by the director of the "National Institute of Diabetes and Digestive and Kidney Disease", Dr. Griffin Rodgers. He said that KIDNEY TRANSPLANT TREATMENT RESEARCH WORK is being done. This remark gives me and people with kidney disease hope for better future. "But some of the barriers for health care is lack of education to the public in general, regarding doses of insulin," he added.

CHAPTER 4

WHAT IS DIABETES?

Many experts have done numerous studies, and all arrive with basically the same conclusion that diabetes is a disease that involves several organs in the body and affects different people in different ways. My goal today, is to discuss some of the research work done by our wonderful experts, educators and World Health Organization {WHO} in their effort to promote awareness of diabetes, treatment, and management of the disease, globally. To understand diabetes, it will be helpful to understand the digestion process, metabolic syndrome, the Somogyi effect vs. Dawn phenomenon theory as related to diabetes.

We get sugar from two sources. In scenario one, glucose is converted from the carbohydrates and starchy food we eat. In scenario two, glucose is manufactured in the liver and muscles.

Digestion process.

The mouth starts the process of food intake. The mouth chews and breaks up the food so it may be passed down the stomach. The stomach and intestines break down the food into nutrients, simpler substances the body can absorb. One of them is simple sugar or glucose. The pancreas produces hormones and substances that help with digestion.

One of these hormones is insulin. The pancreas releases insulin into the blood circulation, which help glucose to enter various cells in the body and be stored. If your body does not make enough insulin, or if the insulin does not work in the way it should, glucose cannot get into the body cells. It stays in your blood, causing your blood glucose level to rise too high. This is called "hyperglycemia". You can compare glucose in your body cells to gasoline in your car. Each is a fuel and a source of energy. If you run out of gasoline in your car, however, it is not enough to make the car move. You also need a key to start the motor, which allows the gasoline to be converted into energy. Like the car, your body also need a key that enables you to use glucose as energy. INSULIN is the key. It opens the cell wall to allow glucose to pass from your blood circulation into the cells, where it produces energy for the body.

Metabolic Syndrome.

Some experts describe metabolic syndrome as a pattern, insulin -resistance syndrome. It is a collection of conditions that when taken together increases the risk of heart disease, stroke and diabetes. Metabolic syndrome is the main deviation from the normal digestive function of the body system. A diagnosis of metabolic syndrome is made if a person has any three of the following risk factors:

> Abdominal obesity or large waist circumference, at least greater than forty {40} inches in men, and greater than thirty-five {35} inches in women; Fasting blood glucose level at least 100mg/Dl ; Serum triglycerides at least 150mg/Dl; Blood pressure at least 135/85mm/Hg; HDL {good} cholesterol lower than 40mg/Dl for men, or 50mg/Dl for women.

L World Health Organization {WHO} emphasizes more on high blood glucose levels, impaired glucose tolerance test, and fasting glucose, as they indicate that the person has diabetes:

Insulin resistance and protein in urine; Urinary albumen secretion ratio of 20mg/minute or higher; Albumin to creatinine ratio/GFR {30mg/minute or higher are also positive factors.

Good attention must be given to the need of prevention and treatment to restore healthy lifestyle. Serious complications always arise in the negative way. Metabolic syndrome appears to affect between 25-30% of the United States population according to various national health surveys. In fact the number of people with metabolic syndrome seems to increase as we get older in our seventies {70's}.

Causes and Symptoms:

Usually there are no immediate physical symptoms. People with metabolic syndrome do have a tendency to be overweight, especially around the abdomen, like an "apple shape". Since the condition is associated with insulin resistance, the individuals with this condition may display some of the clinical symptoms of an increase in the production of insulin. For example, women may experience cysts in their ovaries or irregular menstrual periods, conditions associated with metabolic syndrome. Consistently, high levels of insulin are associated with many harmful changes in the body before its manifestation as a disease.

The cause is unknown. According to experts, it is influenced in most cases by diet and lifestyle. It is also genetically driven. Many features of metabolic syndrome are associated with insulin resistance as well, but the negative result is that it causes the body cells to lose their sensitivity to insulin.

CHAPTER 5

The Somogyi Effect vs. Dawn Phenomenon as related to Diabetes

WebMD-Author Matt Smith also wrote his views on diabetes which was medically reviewed by Michael Dansinger, MD on June 13, 2020.

For people who have diabetes, the Somogyi effect and the dawn phenomenon both cause higher blood sugar levels in the morning. The dawn phenomenon happens naturally, but the Somogyi effect usually happens because of problems with your diabetes management routine, insulin, blood sugar and sleep.

> * Your body uses a form of sugar called glucose as its main source of energy. A hormone, known as insulin, which your pancreas makes, helps your body move glucose from your bloodstream to your cells. While you sleep, your body doesn't need as much energy. But when you're about to wake up, it gets ready to burn more fuel. It tells your liver to start releasing more glucose into your blood. That should trigger your body to release more insulin to handle more blood sugar. If you have diabetes, your body doesn't make enough insulin to

do that. That leaves too much sugar in your blood, a problem called hyperglycemia.

High blood sugar can cause serious health problems, so if you have diabetes, you'll need help to bring those levels down. Diet and exercise help, so can medications like insulin.

Somogyi effect. Cont'd.

Author Anna Schaefer, medically reviewed by Marina Basina, MD. In July 14, 2021. Anna Schaefer shared her view: Somogyi effect happens when you take insulin before bedtime and wake up with high blood sugar levels. This theory explains that when insulin lowers your blood sugar too much, it can trigger release of hormones that send your sugar levels into a rebound high. It is thought to be more common in people with Type- 1 diabetes than Type- 2 diabetes.

Symptoms of the Somogyi effect: You may be experiencing the Somogyi effect if you wake up with high blood sugar levels in the morning, and you don't know why? Night sweats may be a symptom of this theory. Although high glucose in the morning does happen, there is little evidence to support that the Somogyi effect theory is the explanation. But if you notice these symptoms like inconsistencies, or large changes in your blood sugar levels, speak with your doctor.

When you use insulin therapy to control your diabetes, you need to measure your blood sugar levels several times a day. Depending on the results, you might take insulin to lower your blood sugar levels, or have a snack to raise them.

CHAPTER 6

The Dawn phenomenon

Dawn phenomenon experience is similar to the Somogyi effect, but the causes are different. Every experiences, the Dawn phenomenon to some extent, it's your body's natural response to hormones cortisol, growth hormone and catecholamine that are released as morning approaches. These hormones trigger the release of glucose from your liver. In most people the release of glucose is tempered by the release of insulin. But if you have diabetes, your body doesn't release more insulin to match the early morning rise in blood sugar. It's called the dawn phenomenon, since it usually happens between 3a.m. and 8a.m. in the morning. The dawn phenomenon happens to nearly everyone with diabetes, but there are a few ways to prevent it, including:

1. Don't eat carbohydrates before going to bed.
2. Take insulin before bedtime instead of earlier in the evening.
3. Ask your doctor about adjusting your dose of insulin or other diabetes medicines.
4. Use an insulin pump overnight.

How Do You Know Which One You Have?

Your doctor will want to find out why you're waking up with high blood sugar before they tell you how to treat it. This means they'll ask you to test your blood sugar in the middle of the night- around 2-3 a.m. - for several nights.

If your levels are always low during that time, it's probably the somogyi effect. If not, it's likely the dawn phenomenon. Knowing which is which will help your doctor come up with a plan to address it. The underlying cause of diabetes varies by type.

CHAPTER 7

Diabetes- Symptoms and Causes – Mayo Clinic

Diabetes mellitus refers to a group of diseases that affect how your body uses blood sugar {glucose}. Glucose is vital to your health because it's an important source of energy for the cells that make up your muscles and tissues. It's also your brain's main source of fuel. The underlying cause of diabetes varies by type. But, no matter what type of diabetes you have, it can lead to excess sugar in your blood. Diabetes symptoms vary depending on how much your blood sugar is elevated .Some people, especially those with prediabetes or Type-2 diabetes may sometimes experience symptoms. In Type-1 diabetes, symptoms tend to come quickly and be more severe. Some of the signs and symptoms of Type-1 diabetes and Type-2 diabetes are:

1. Increased thirst
2. Frequent urination.
3. Extreme hunger.
4. Unexplained weight loss.

CHAPTER 8

Diabetes Myths and Misconceptions

Several myths. Cultural beliefs, poverty, and lack of education may contribute to the fear and apprehension about living with diabetes and the fact that the disease will shorten your life, considering all the complications it entails. These statements might discourage you but there is help for learning to overcome the barriers. This topic will be Q&A. format.

1. Can you develop diabetes by eating sugar?
    Many people get confused when they hear this question, but the experts say that eating too much sugar will not cause diabetes. But people with diabetes have to watch for the total number of calories on their plate. What is calorie? It is the measurement of fuel or energy value of food. If you eat excessive calories of any kind, causing you to gain weight and develop insulin resistance, you may end up with diabetes. American Diabetes Association {ADA} recommends that a healthy diet may include up to 15% of its caloric content from simple sugar so long as the other 85% is obtained from a healthy distribution of fats, proteins and carbohydrates. For example, you may not add sugar to your beverage but will eat a lot of fats and starchy foods. It is better for a diabetic to eat whole grain, leafy vegetables, and drink more water.

2. Is Insulin number one therapy for diabetes?

    Insulin therapy can be avoided. Some experts may agree that there are many alternatives to having to inject yourself more often. Insulin is not addictive, and it is not given as a drug. Insulin is used as a replacement therapy for the naturally occurring hormone "insulin". In a safer side, sometimes it is used in pregnancy, in some cases of infection, heart attack, or major surgical procedures. People may need insulin temporarily to control their sugar levels. This does not mean in those circumstances, that you will be on insulin the rest of your life. Actually, early treatment of insulin therapy may prevent diabetes complications, such as kidney failure, heart disease, eyes and nerve damage. Good blood pressure and cholesterol levels are positive outcome of insulin therapy. On the negative side, insulin therapy can be time consuming and demanding of a person's attention than exercise, diet control, medication, and managing diabetes itself.

3. Can Women with Diabetes nave Children, or should They Not have Children?

    There might be women who are afraid to have children because of misconception and belief system in the society. People with diabetes can have children if they want. For example, I have children, and I am living with diabetes. I will tell my audience that there are some risks involved. Women with poorly controlled diabetes during pregnancy may experience problems. Some women are diagnosed with "gestational diabetes" during pregnancy, which puts both mother and the baby into complications during pregnancy, labor and delivery. Some women recover after post- partum or delivery of the baby. But there is high risk for developing Type-2 diabetes later on in life. Read more on the subsequent chapter of "Types of Diabetes", for more information on this topic.

CHAPTER 9

Types of Diabetes

Prediabetes: This is an early warning sign of metabolic syndrome that can lead to developing Type- 2 diabetes. The good news is that maintaining a healthy weight and being physically active can often reverse the condition and delay or prevent the development of Type-2 diabetes. You need medical supervision from the health –care team and set your goal to live a healthy lifestyle. You need to be screened for the warning signs or the risk factors for prediabetes, which are as follows:

1. Are you overweight? Studies show that being overweight alone contributes more than fifty percent {50%} risk factor for developing diabetes, more so without physical activity, while inactive lean women risk double to develop diabetes.
2. Do you have excess weight around your waist?
3. Is your diet high in carbohydrates, such as white bread, potatoes, and pasta?
4. Do you eat starchy snack food or sweets?
5. Do you exercise less than three {3} hours per week?
6. Are you African-American, Hispanic American, Native American, Asian American, or Pacific Islander? They have higher risk for developing diabetes with high mortality rate.
7. Do you have any family history of diabetes, including father, mother, brother or sister?"

8. Do you have increased blood pressure/ hypertension readings of over 140/90 mm/Hg?
9. Do you have high triglyceride?
10. Are you over forty-five {45} years old?

High blood sugar/glucose levels over months and years in most cases can lead to serious complications. For most people, the higher the blood sugar level, the higher the chance of complications. Extremely high blood sugar levels can cause loss of consciousness and even death. Overall, the risk of death is twice as high with people with diabetes rather than those without the disease. Therefore, you should pay attention to screening and prevention of diabetes and its complications. I strongly encourage anyone, or your family member with any risk factor, to get your screening tests done without hesitation.

CHAPTER 10

Type-1 Diabetes

For some people with diabetes, insulin is not able to carry out its function for one of two reasons: The pancreas may not produce enough insulin, and this is known as Type-1 diabetes. In some cases, the pancreas is no longer producing insulin and this is why Type-1 is also called insulin dependent diabetes mellitus {IDDM}. In Type-1, the specialized beta cells of the pancreas stop producing insulin. The condition usually starts in childhood, and people who are diagnosed with the disease require lifelong insulin therapy and careful dietary management to survive. Recently, stem cell - transplants have been successful also for the treatment of Type-1 diabetes. Most of Type-1 cases are caused by auto -immune disease. The body mistakenly attacks and destroys the beta cells in the pancreas that produce insulin. Type-1 diabetes strikes suddenly. You may appear fine one day, and be very sick just a few weeks or days later.

CHAPTER 11

Type-2 Diabetes

In general, whenever we talk about diabetes, we are referring to Type-2 diabetes. About 90- 95% or even probably higher today, of people diagnosed with diabetes have Type-2, a disease that is quite different from Type-1. In a large majority of cases, the individual still makes insulin. In fact, the person may make large amounts of insulin, but the body cells respond more slowly to its presence. This condition is also known as insulin resistance. Over time, with this slow response of the cell to the insulin signal, the rising of blood sugar/glucose levels become above normal range. This process may seem difficult to understand and figure out what is going on in your body. But what we see here simply explains how insulin tries to knock hard at the cell walls and signals to the cell for blood glucose/sugar to enter. There is resistance at this juncture, because the cell walls do not open, leading to high glucose levels in the blood stream. This is known as "Hyperglycemia".

At this stage, the pancreas pours more insulin into the blood circulation to force glucose to enter the cells. If the pancreas is able to perform this function but the cell walls may not allow sufficient sugar/glucose to enter, the individual becomes hypoglycemic, or he /she will have low glucose levels in the blood stream. This problem causes lots of damage to the body organs. As time goes on, the pancreas fails to produce enough insulin at such high levels, and this is why "insulin" must be administered in order to control the blood sugar levels.

CHAPTER 12

Children with Type-2 Diabetes

Type-2 diabetes was primarily a problem for older people. It was not common to find children and people in their twenties {20+ years}, with Type-2 diabetes. Today, even children are being diagnosed with this disease. About forty- five percent {45 %} of children with nearly diagnosed diabetes have Type- 2, according to some research report. One in every three children born in the year 2000 developed diabetes, which is still affecting more children today. To prevent increase in this report, and for diabetes management in general, we all must work to support the goals established by "World Health Organization {WHO}". The emphasis must be focus on:

1. Promoting healthy diets globally.
2. Preventing and controlling non- communicable diseases like diabetes.
3. Maintaining a healthy lifestyle, exercising for weight loss, sports activities in schools and fitness centers etc.
4. Encourage multimedia- Education.
5. Access to diabetes treatment and management are encouraged, with medical supervision.

CHAPTER 13

Polycystic Ovary Syndrome

Like all risk factors for Type-2 diabetes, there is evidence of increased insulin resistance and even increased insulin secretion by the pancreas. Hormonal imbalance can cause irregular menstrual periods, infertility, weight gain, and excessive hair growth. About eleven percent {11%} of women diagnosed with polycystic ovary syndrome are between the ages of twenty and twenty-five {20-25} years old. Treatment includes diet control for diabetes in general, and follow all the guidelines established by World Health Organization {WHO}.

Gestational Diabetes.

About forty percent {40 %} of pregnant women each year in the United States of America develop gestational diabetes. Risk factors can be related to the following:

1. Women over twenty- five {25} years who are obese with any of the following:
   - Increased blood sugar levels/hyperglycemia.
   - Increased blood pressure/hypertension
   - Family history of diabetes.
   - Belonging to certain ethnic groups.

The problematic outcome with gestational diabetes may be an infant with increased birth weight, which causes difficulty during labor and delivery, including possibility of caesarean section. Risks to infants include high concentration of glucose levels in their blood before birth to the first few days postpartum. Breathing problem is most likely to occur and may require oxygen therapy if baby is born early. Baby may become overweight and develop diabetes later because of inheriting mother's metabolic tendencies. To control gestational diabetes, we must be proactive and adopt a healthy lifestyle forever by paying particular attention to the following needs:

1. Diet plan suitable for all diabetes individuals.
2. Sensible exercise during pregnancy.
3. Monitor your blood glucose levels frequently, and know your lows and highs so you can treat those warning signs.
   Blood glucose levels usually return to normal after delivery. However, about twenty to fifty percent {20- 50%} chance of developing Type-2 diabetes within the next few years is possible.

CHAPTER 14

Overview of Type-1 and Type-2 Diabetes

	Type 1	**Type 2**
Characteristics - oral	Insulin dependent	May or may not need insulin, medication
Age	Begins before age 20- 40+	Occurs in all age groups.
Insulin	Little or none produced, insulin may not be enough.	Pancreas produces insulin.
Onset	Sudden.	Slow.
Gender	Both males and females.	More females are affected.
Heredity	Some tendency.	Strong tendency.
Weight	Majority are thin/ weight loss.	Overweight.
Ketones	Ketones present in urine.	No ketone in urine.
Treatment - oral	Insulin, diet, exercise.	Diet, exercise, insulin, medication.

CHAPTER 15

A. What happens if Diabetes is left untreated?

Left untreated, both types of diabetes lead to complications that damage your cardiovascular system, kidney and nerves due to high blood glucose/ sugar levels.

Complications due to untreated diabetes such as ketoacidosis are fatal, if not treated.

B. What are the signs and symptoms of uncontrolled Diabetes?

* Uncontrolled diabetes is defined by "Sandra Parker" in the year 2017, as a condition where the body either doesn't produce enough insulin, or the cells have become resistant to insulin: Ether way, the body isn't able to make use of glucose.in the bloodstream, so the cells begin to die, and tissue damage occurs.

* Signs and Symptoms of uncontrolled - diabetes are:

— Frequent urination, unusual thirst, weight loss, hunger, changes in vision,
— Lethargy, sores that do not heal may turn to
— Ulcers, tingling sensation in the hands and feet.

C. What are the long term effects of untreated Diabetes?

The most common long term diabetes- related health problems are:

1. Damage to the small blood vessels causing problems in the eyes, kidneys, feet and nerves {microvascular complications}.
2. Damage to the large blood vessels of your heart, brain and legs {macrovascular complications}.

CHAPTER 16

KIDNEY DISEASE

Stage 3 of Chronic Kidney Disease:

A person with stage 3 chronic kidney disease {CKD} has moderate kidney damage. This stage is broken up into two : a decrease in glomerular filtration rate {GFR} for Stage 3A is 45-59mL/min and a decrease in GFR for Stage 3B is 30-44mL/min. As kidney function declines waste products can build up in the blood causing a condition known as "uremia". In stage 3, a person is more likely to develop complications of kidney disease such as, high blood pressure, anemia{a shortage of red blood cells} and /or early bone disease. Many people who develop CKD have diabetes or high blood pressure. By keeping their glucose level under control and maintaining a healthy blood pressure, this can help them preserve their kidney function. As stage 3 progresses, a patient should see a nephrologist {a doctor who specializes in treating kidney disease} for proper management.

SYMPTOMS OF STAGE 3 CKD.

The symptoms may start to become present in Stage 3:
* **Fatigue**
* **Fluid retention, swelling {edema} of extremities and shortness osf breath.**

* Urination changes {foaming; dark orange, brown, tea-colored or red if it contains blood; and urinating more or less than normal}.
* Kidney pain felt in their back.
* Sleep problem due to muscle clamps or restless legs.
*   MEETING A DIETITIAN WHEN YOU HAVE STAGE 3 CKD: As stated before in my book cover summary, someone in Stage 3 CKD may also be referred to a dietitian. Because diet is such an important part of treatment, the dietician will review a person's lab work results and recommend a meal plan suitable and individualized for their needs. Eating a proper diet can help preserve kidney function and overall health.

For Stage 3 CKD, A healthy diet is likely to consist of:

* Eating high- quality protein and potassium {if blood levels are above normal}.
* Consuming some grains, fruits and vegetables {potassium and phosphorus are at normal levels}.
* limiting phosphorus to help PTH levels remain normal, prevent bone disease and even preserve existing kidney function.
* Lowering calcium consumption.
* Cutting back carbohydrates for those with diabetes.
* Decreasing saturated fats to help lower cholesterol.
* Lowering sodium for people with high blood pressure or fluid retention by cutting out processed and pre-packaged foods.
* Limiting calcium if blood levels are too high.
* Taking water soluble vitamins such as C {100mg per day} and B-Complex, or completely avoiding over the –counter dietary supplements unless approved by the nephrologist}.

CHAPTER 17

Treatment for End-stage kidney disease

More often kidney function worsens over a number of years. This is called chronic kidney disease {CKD} until there is less than ten percent {10 %} function left. The condition then becomes what is known as end-stage kidney disease or kidney failure. This is when kidney replacement therapy is needed. People with kidney failure need dialysis or kidney transplant to stay alive. Together, the two treatments are known as "Kidney Replacement Therapy." Dialysis is temporary for some people with acute renal failure. They have this treatment until their kidneys begin to work again.

*My focus today in this chapter is Kidney Dialysis treatment for end stage kidney disease. So your doctor will order routine urine testing for presence of protein and monitor your blood pressure levels vigorously. You may need to take special medications to protect your kidneys.

The good news is that eating vegetarian source of protein and less amount of it on your plate might be good for your kidneys. So when a person with chronic kidney disease {CKD} reaches Stage-5 kidney disease or kidney failure, or end stage renal disease, the kidneys are no longer functioning to filter and clean the blood the way healthy kidneys normally would. Life without treatment will cause waste and toxins to build up in the body. At this point, dialysis treatment, or a kidney transplant is needed to prolong life.

Dialysis Treatment.

When kidneys fail, your body may have difficulty cleaning your blood and keeping your system chemically balanced. Dialysis can take the place of some kidney function, and along with medication, and proper care help people live longer. Dialysis is a treatment for kidney failure that rids your body of unwanted toxins, waste products and excess fluids by filtering your blood. Dialysis treatment is prescribed by your doctor. Together, you and your doctor will discuss treatment options and determine what's right for you. If YOU DECIDE TO GO ON DIALYSIS, your doctor will prescribe your treatment time and frequency, based on your unique health needs. IT'S IMPORTANT TO COMPLETE YOUR DIALYSIS TREATMENT exactly as prescribed. Before dialysis, classes are given to the patients for encouragement so they can feel their best when on dialysis. The patients can even choose the class format that fits their life. Classes are educator- led or self-guided, to prepare you for dialysis. The doctors do a number of lab tests, such as kidney function tests when determining treatment.

Types of Dialysis.

There are two types of dialysis: **Hemodialysis and Peritoneal dialysis.** Depending on which type of dialysis you choose, you may also have options for treating in a center, or at home.

1. Hemodialysis filter your blood through dialysis machine. The filtering membrane is called "Dialyzer", and is inside a dialysis machine. Solution used for dialysis is called DIALYSATE for the filtering process to remove unwanted substances from your bloodstream. Your blood is circulated through the dialysis machine, and cleaned before being returned to your body. Once

you are connected to the machine via your hemodialysis access, blood flows into the machine, gets filtered and is returned to your body. There is a choice in where you do hemodialysis and who performs the treatment. "In- center hemodialysis" is performed by a trained team of nurses and technicians.

"At- home hemodialysis" can be performed in the comfort of your own home, either with the help of a care partner or on your own.

2. Peritoneal dialysis: This dialysis uses the blood vessels in the lining of your stomach, the body's natural filter, along with a solution called "Dialysate" to filter blood via a peritoneal catheter. With this method, blood never leaves your body. Peritoneal dialysis can be done with a machine or manually at home, at work or even while traveling.

Summary:

*   Treatment options for kidney failure include dialysis, kidney transplantation or supportive care
*   There are two types of dialysis- peritoneal dialysis and hemodialysis.
*   Dialysis can be performed at home, which is less disruptive.to lifestyle and may have health benefits.
*   Kidney transplant is a treatment for kidney failure, not a cure.
*   Some people choose supportive care rather than dialysis or kidney transplantation.

CHAPTER 18

SOME PROBLEMS RELATED
TO DIABETES

Aside complications of DIABETES, such as stroke, heart attack, kidney failure, leg amputation, retinopathy, etc. there are other problems related to diabetes, if untreated can cause serious damage to your body functions, and it is important to learn which are these, so that you can pay attention to the warning signs seriously to prevent any negative outcome, especially if you have family history of diabetes.

1. Nerve Damage:

People with diabetes are at risk for nerve damage, which can take two forms. "Peripheral Neuropathy" is sometimes called sensorimotor neuropathy, which indicates the damage to the nerves that allows you to feel things or to move your muscles. It leads to tingling sensation, pain, numbness or weakness in your feet or hands. It pays to take these signs seriously, because although it can get better, it can also get a lot worse if you are not careful.

2. Immune System:

Too much blood glucose levels can also hinder the immune system's function of fighting white blood cells {WBC}, making you more vulnerable to illnesses. Reduced sensation in your feet can make you vulnerable to injuries that you cannot feel. It is easy to overlook a small cut or scrape, when you do not feel it. Injuries that you think are healed can set you up for festering infection. Leg amputation and poor wound healing become a major financial and emotional burden on the individual, regardless of his or her immobility. The family and the society as a whole suffer as well, emotionally and financially. Dear reader, my own uncle had "bilateral above- knee amputation." He died some few years ago. As a nurse, I was challenged to play a major role in his care.

Autonomic Neuropathy:

This is abnormalities in the nerves that control your internal functions. It can lead to digestive problems such as nausea, vomiting, constipation or diarrhea. It can cause problems in the bladder control, or sexual function. Other symptoms include dizziness, fainting episodes, increased or decreased sweating, visual problems adjusting to light and dark conditions. There may be lack of awareness if there is a warning sign of "hypoglycemia." The key to prevention and treatment of neuropathy is to control your diabetes.

3. Eye Problems:

Your eyes are delicate cameras that capture the world around you, transmitting their details to your brain to perceive and remember. In the same way that a camera is fragile, several parts of the eye are susceptible to damage. High blood pressure, high blood glucose levels, and high cholesterol levels increase your risk of developing eye conditions like glaucoma, cataract, and retinopathy, leading to blindness. The increased pressure in the eye pinches on the tiny blood vessels on the retina and the optic nerve. Millions of tiny nerves in the retina, which is located at the back of the eye just like a camera film, become damaged, leading to retinopathy. The tiny blood capillaries balloon out and leak substances into the retina, leading to the formation of fatty deposits. For some time, the blood vessels begin to bleed and cause scarring. Your best defense is to get the risk factors under control, and have eye examinations done by an ophthalmologist, at least once a year. I had major eye surgery in the year 2011. The cataract, known as " opacity of the lens", affected my both eyes. The end result was that I had the cataracts in both eyes extracted and replaced with inplant lenses. Few years later, I was diagnosed with glaucoma in both eyes. Today, I put eye drops on my eyes daily for glaucoma. I thank God for such intervention to help many people survive because of new medical interventions arriving in today's market.

4.   Sleep Apnea And Diabetes:

It is very common to see some people diagnosed with metabolic syndrome experiencing this problem. Feeling tired in the morning after waking up can explain that you may have sleep apnea with a sleep -related breathing disorder.

Signs and symptoms:

Your breathing stops or becomes very shallow as you sleep. This is called "Obstructive Sleep Apnea {OSA}, which is frequently diagnosed. Most times your breathing may pause for some minutes. It occurs when the soft tissue in the back of the throat relaxes and blocks the passage of air until your airway opens, with a loud choking or gasping sound, and you begin to breathe again. Other signs and symptoms of sleep apnea include snoring loudly, Getting your sleep apnea diagnosed and treated will help you get a good sleep at night.{Studies show that 5% of diagnosed individuals snore loudly}. If you have a large neck, the size of your neck can be a positive sign for sleep apnea, as well as being overweight {according to statistics women with OSA have a neck size of sixteen centimeters {16cm} or more, while men have seventeen centimeters {17 cm} or more. Another sign is that you wake up frequently for bathroom breaks. Check with your doctor if you have any of these risk factors for proper evaluation and treatment.

CHAPTER 19

SELF- MANAGEMENT FOR DIABETES IS NECESSARY AT ALL TIMES

Lab -works:

Your doctor may order the following laboratory tests for diagnostic purposes during routine visits:

1. *Complete Blood Count {CBC}: This test shows the state of your blood cells. Many people with diabetes develop anemia, meaning they have fewer red blood cells than they should. If your CBC is low, your doctor will investigate the reasons for it, which could include kidney disease, iron deficiency anemia, use of certain medications, and abnormal bleeding.

2. * Urine Testing-Fast Fact: The first glucose monitor was invented in India thousands of years ago. A physician would spill a sample of patient's urine unto the ground then study how fast ants would crawl toward the urine spot. Thus he would be able to judge how high the patient's sugars were. Urine test are still the method used to check the ketones in urine. When insulin levels are extremely low in people with Type-1 diabetes, the body turns to fat for sources of energy and produces ketones. This usually indicates that the person's blood sugar levels are

extremely high, and the individual is said to be in ketoacidosis. Patients may be advised by their doctors to check their urine for ketones if their sugar levels are running above 250-300mg/Dl consistently. Today, some blood pressure monitors also check ketones in the blood. Generally, your doctor should check your urine every six – twelve months for protein excretion. Presence of albumin in urine may be an early sign of kidney disease.

3. Fasting Plasma Glucose {FPG} or Casual plasma glucose test: To confirm the diagnosis of Type-2 diabetes, your doctor will order a casual plasma glucose test.

   This is a preferred method for diagnosing diabetes, because it is easy to do, convenient, and less expensive than tests, according to American Diabetes Association {ADA}. The patient should fast at least eight{8} hours prior to the test. Blood is drawn and sent to the laboratory for analysis. The result of 70- 100mg/Dl, is normal for nondiabetics. When your readings for two separate fasting blood glucose levels are greater than or equal to 126mg/Dl, it indicates you are a diabetic.

4. *Hemoglobin A1C: This blood test helps you and your doctor understand how well your treatment plan is working within every three months period. For many people with diabetes, A1C of less than 7% is a good goal. If your test result is 7% or more, you need your doctor to change your treatment plan, since your blood sugar is not well controlled. Each person has unique needs and goals.

*Reference: {What is A1C Mayo Clinic?}.

The A1C test is common blood test used to diagnosed Type-1 and Type-2 diabetes and to monitor how well you're managing you're managing your diabetes. The A1C test goes by many other names, including glycated hemoglobin, glycosylated hemoglobin, hemoglobin

A1C and HbA1c. The A1C test result reflects your average blood sugar levels for the past three months.

5. *Glucose Tolerance Test {GTT}:

Is your FPT is normal but you show some signs of risk factors, the doctor may order this test.

The reasons are that blood sugar rises rapidly as you eat or impaired glucose intolerance. If your

Blood sugar levels are high enough, you may be diagnosed with diabetes. GTT is a time consuming and expensive test, but it is the best way the body reacts to carbohydrate intake.

CHAPTER 20

HOME MANAGEMENT ACTIVITIES

It is important to wear "Diabetic Bracelet," for emergencies or carry an emergency card in your wallet, including medication lists on the card, your doctor's and family's contact information with name, phone number, etc. Carry remedy food, candies, soda with carb-source with you to quickly manage low blood sugar levels.

Questions To Ask Yourself:

1. Is your blood sugar/glucose levels within the recommended range?
2. Are any of your numbers under or over your recommended target?
3. Do you notice any daily pattern?
4. Are there times during the day that your blood sugar/glucose level is higher than target range?
5. Can you think of any reason why your blood glucose/sugar acted as it did?

Sample of DAILY Blood sugar/glucose Profile:

Day 1.
When tested? Before breakfast.
Time of day? 7: a.m.
Blood sugar test result {mg/dL.}? = 120mg/dL

If you have been managing your diabetes well, eating well, exercising, and taking your medication, and your morning blood sugar test result is still high, you may be going to bed with your blood sugar level within the target range, but your levels are high in the morning. Please refer to the "Dawn phenomenon theory." To correct this, your doctor may base on the results of your blood testing throughout the night or recommend you not to eat carbohydrates close to bedtime. Adjusting your dose of medication or insulin, or switching you to a different medication are other options of intervention.

Restful Sleep:

Recharge your energy with restful sleep. If you frequently toss and turn at night, you will be tired during the day. Try to create a friendly environment for good sleep. Wear loose, comfortable clothes. Check your blood sugar levels more than once, because high or low levels can affect the quality of your sleep. If your sugar level is low, eat some snack. Inform your doctor of any unusual levels or pattern. Determine and use good night time routine that relaxes your body, and help you to sleep. Fight insomnia with sleep tactics. Be drowsy or sleepy before going to bed. For example, some people read stories, watch movies or listen to favorite music. Refreshing sleep, deep, daily serenity are good for you. Get extra support from family members or by other means if you are feeling burned out with children and home chores. Get real help if you are depressed. Taking care of your disease is a choice you make right now and forever.

CHAPTER 21

Exercise, diet and weight loss

Exercise can help you lose weight and keep it off for better outcome. It is very difficult to exercise enough to lose without also changing what you eat. Adding aerobic or cardiovascular exercise to your routine is best for weight loss. This is a kind of exercise that gets your heart pumping. Walking, jogging, bicycling, swimming, and dancing, all can help you to lose weight, because they are the large muscles in your body that burn the most calories. You can walk by yourself or with company. Walking is safer than jogging or running, and puts less stress on your body. It is good choice if you have been sedentary or have joint or balance problem. If you walk to visit friends, shop and do household chore, then you can probably walk for exercise. Using a cane or walker need not stop you from walking routine. Your goal is to walk most days of the week, at your pace, then increase the intensity at a time and do the best you can. Exercising in the evening may help keep morning blood sugar levels in a better range.

*Effect of exercises for your body:

Good exercises help to lower blood sugar levels, especially in people with Type- 2 diabetes. Transformation from prediabetes to Type-2 diabetes or even to insulin dependence can be prevented. Exercise can reduce adipose tissue in your body. It can lower insulin levels enabling your body cells to respond to insulin properly. There is improvement in Cholesterol level, triglycerides, as well as other lipid levels, and blood pressure is controlled. Attaining proper weight for your frame is enhanced by exercising regularly. Exercising improves mental alertness, it is stress relief mechanism, promotes stronger immunity from diseases.

*Diet for Diabetes:

*Best food to control diabetes: Reference :{mayo clinic.org; healthline. com}.

Gallic, broccoli, Fish, such as salmon, sardines, herring, anchovies and mackerel are all good source of omega-3 fatty acids.

*Wrong foods to eat are potato, pasta, carbohydrates, soda, cookies, sweet candy, etc.

*What is the best diet plan for diabetics to lose weight?

American Diabetes Association {ADA} says diabetic meal plan often contain the following:

1. Three meals and two snacks daily.
2. The best diet for diabetic to lose weight consist of a regular meal plan, reduced calorie intake, and a controlled carbohydrate intake.

*Reference: {health fully.com/435427-the-best-diabetic-diet-for-weight-loss.com}.

CHAPTER 22

MOTIVATION

1. Coping Mechanism:

How people respond to stress is different from each other, depending on what type of stress, how you handled similar stress in the past or your ability to solve problems. It is not easy all the time, but I encourage you to be positive and do your best. You are strong and a winner. Pay attention to some risk factors, such as sudden illness, traveling, work-related stress, marriage or sudden death in the family. Try also to deal with stress in a more therapeutic way, such as counseling therapy, so you can learn how to stay motivated to manage diabetes, and stay happy with a new attitude in life.

2. Consistency:

Being consistent from day to day, when it comes to diet and exercise is the key to managing diabetes. Over time, you as an individual will have lots of things to do in life as a human being. You want to work, get married, travel or have children. These are facts of life, and is a good feeling. From time to time as your routine changes, you will face challenges that can affect your blood glucose, and other aspects of your health. But be consistent, believe in yourself, that having the ability to manage certain circumstances in your life is an invaluable skill.

3. Perseverance:

Perseverance will pay off as you work hard to manage your diabetes, or take care of your love ones. Learn to take full control of your disease, don't hesitate to get help if necessary. Work closely with your doctor and the health- care team for medical supervision. Persevere to fight against diabetes, your goal is to live a healthy lifestyle and at the end you will know that your blood glucose levels are within normal range.

Take your medications and do laboratory tests, as ordered by your health-care providers. One of the unique features of exercise is re-gaining your health is entirely up to you. You may put exercise at the bottom of the list for diabetes control despite all the benefits. Diabetes management is individualized. The choice of food, amount of calories on your plate, time of day you eat, activities, weight, stress level, medication you take, etc., all affect blood sugar/glucose levels and insulin function in your body. It is possible to reverse the bad readings to desired levels or values. Adopting a healthy lifestyle is a good decision for a diabetic to make. Maintain a positive attitude that will help you to control your diabetes.

CHAPTER 23

Statistics about Diabetes

American Diabetes Association studies have found that only about 35-40% of people with diabetes who died had diabetes listed anywhere on the death certificate, and about 10- 15% had it listed as the underlying cause of death. Diabetes was the seventh leading cause of death in the United States in 2017, based on the death certificates in which diabetes was listed as the underlying cause of death. In 2017, diabetes was mentioned as a cause of death in a total of 270, 702 certificates.

Overall Numbers:

- **Prevalence:** In 2018, 34.2 million Americans, or 10.5% of the population, had diabetes.

   Nearly 1.6 million Americans have Type-1 diabetes, including about 187,000 children, and adolescents.

***Undiagnosed: Of the 34.2 million adults with diabetes, 26.8 million were diagnosed, and 7.3 million were undiagnosed.**
***Prevalence in Seniors: The percentage of Americans age 65 and older remain in high at 26.8%, or 14.3 million seniors {diagnosed and undiagnosed}.**

*New cases: 1.5 million Americans are diagnosed with diabetes every year.
*Prediabetes: In 2015, 88 million Americans age 18 and older had prediabetes.

Diabetes by Race/ Ethnicity.

*The rates of diagnosed diabetes in adults by race/ethnic background are:

1. 7.5% of non- Hispanic whites.
2. 9.2% of Asian Americans.
3. 12.5% of Hispanics.
4. 11.7% of non- Hispanic blacks.
5. 14.7% of American Indians/ Alaskan Natives.

CHAPTER 24

REFERENCES

- World Health Organization {WHO} –Global reports on diabetes. {www.Bing.com}.
- C-SPAN- U.S.A.- Diabetes Research Report in July, 2019.
- Kidney beginnings. by the American Association of kidney Patients. {www.aakp.org} Genetic Alliance, reprinted 2015, - Tampa-FL, U.S.A.
- www.bing.com/search?/q=kidneydialysis+treatment.
- Davita. Kidney care.
- Kidney dialysis treatment/Better Health Channel:

www.betterhealth.vic.gov.au/healthconditionstreatments/kidneys-dialysis.

- Diabetes- symptoms and causes.{www.mayoclinic.org}.
- What is A1C Mayo Clinic? {www.mayoclinic.org}
- https://www.davita.com/education/kidney disease
- www.bing.com/search?q=ACE+andARB+MEDICATIONS
- Diabetes Research Report in July, 2019- C-SPAN FORUM on Television.
- Diabetes Education-Mayo clinic- {www.mayo clinic.org}
- Reverse diabetes Forever BY Readers Digest Association, INC, New York.

- Mosby's pocket dictionary of medicine, nursing, & Allied health, 1990, C.V. Mosby company, St-Louis-U.S.A. Kenneth N. Anderson & Lois E. Anderson.
  *ADA- Connected for Life.
  {www.diabetes.org/resources/statistics-about -diabetes}.